“Just because everything is different, doesn’t mean anything has changed.”

–Irene Peter

Changeless Change

Manufactured in the United States of America

www.ChangelessChange.com

Have you ever felt like everyone has a rule book but you?

How many years have you spent trying to figure out this thing called life?

How long have you been looking for the rule book?

Are you just about at the end of your rope, ready to give up?

Are you tired? Angry?

Tired of being angry with everyone and everything?

Feel like you don't fit in this world?

Stop!

Hang on!

Look no further.

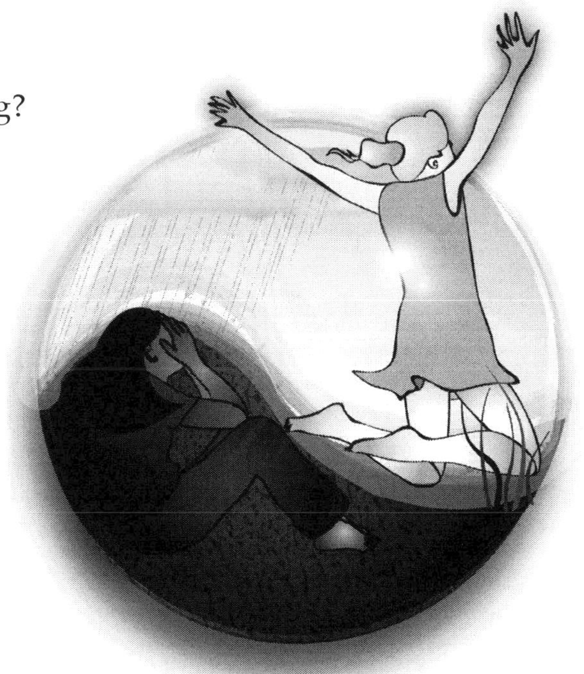

You are holding in your hands *The* Rule Book,

Changeless Change.

It is a map out of the darkness, into the light.

TABLE OF CONTENTS

Foreword

When I was in Al-Anon, we were invited to turn our lives around by eliminating old thoughts and behaviors that no longer worked for us. I wondered, "If I let go of the old me, what will happen? Who will I be—Swiss cheese with big holes where resentment and guilt used to be?" In Changeless Change, Carol Davis provides the answer.

In guiding us from the dark side of ourselves into the positive, light side of ourselves, we don't lose anything. In fact, we find the real person we were meant to be. We were not born to feel like victims, separate from everyone else, or to play small because we don't have the confidence to step out of our comfort zone. There's a whole side to each of us that is bright, shining, and courageous, just waiting for us to notice it! Now is the time. This book leads the way.

What a blessing to have found someone like Carol Davis who reminds us we each bring our unique gifts to the world. Don't worry if you don't know what your gifts are; in the suggestions and exercises offered in Changeless Change they will begin to be uncovered, and you will step out into your life in such a way that your gifts will shine.

Carol's wisdom invites us to trust ourselves and the process. As we choose to see the world from a fresh perspective, new roots of positivity will take hold in the recesses of our minds and hearts, getting ready to sprout as joyous, fulfilling experiences.

Oh, Great Spirit, open the door to my heart and soul.

Release the truth within me

Waiting to be felt

To be heard

To be seen.

Welcome to the journey of self-discovery, opening the door to your heart and soul, releasing the truth within you.

Very gratefully,

Rev. Jane Beach

Author of *Immortality ~ Facing Death with Hope and Peace*

Introduction

All those years I spent running around the world looking for The Rule Book, I thought I was looking for someone to teach me how to live life. I believe many people did, in fact, try to teach me, but I could not hear. Ultimately, I discovered I didn't listen to them because what I was really looking for was someone or something to fix me.

This book, *Changeless Change,* is about knowing I am the problem and I am the answer. Every idea I present here has worked (and still works) for me. I appreciate uncomplicated, pragmatic answers; pages and pages of psychobabble never helped me.

When I discovered I was not the only person feeling what I was feeling I did enjoy some merits from counseling; it is a great comfort to know others experience similar issues. But for those readers who believe their case is different, I understand. I also waved the "I stand alone" flag, and for that reason, I will offer to you a short summary of my journey.

I was relentless in my pursuit of The Rule Book. I never stayed anywhere or with anyone for too long. If I didn't find "it" wherever I was within six months, maximum, I moved on. I had 28 jobs in five states in 11 years. I was chased by police in five countries and arrested in a communist country. I was beaten repeatedly and left to die in gutters around the world, but I kept looking. My life was in a downward spiral, but I kept searching. I always felt that in the next town, or with a new job, or in my next relationship, someone would show me how to live.

About nine years into this 11-year odyssey, my grandmother gave me a house in a suburb of Boston. I believed this would be the answer to all my problems, so I packed my knapsack with all my belongings and headed east for a new beginning. I still had not learned that wherever I go, I take me with me. So, of course, my life continued to spiral downward.

Several years after moving into my house, I was near the end of my search. I could not go on. I attempted suicide, to no avail. I beat up my house, put holes in the walls, broke dishes. One day I had had enough. Even though I lived alone, I ran away from home. I "moved" to the streets, living in a park known as Boston Commons. I actually enjoyed my time there, sleeping on park benches and eating out of garbage cans. I had long given up hope of ever finding The Rule Book and now no creditors or other well-meaning people could bug me about "getting my life together" and other such absurdities. Didn't they know I never got a fair shake because I didn't know how? And besides that, I did not ask to be born anyway. I was pretty well convinced I was not the problem. It was people, places and things; it was anything, or anyone, other than me—I was certain. I had tried so hard for so long and I was so very tired. I even began to think my problem was that I am an Aquarian; perhaps the world was just not ready for me yet.

One day I wandered into a building where coffee and donuts were being served. I was told that if I wanted to eat I would need to wait until the end of whatever it was they were doing. All I wanted was coffee, but I soon found I would be given much more. As I drank my coffee, my "band of angels" (as I now call them) told me if I followed them they would teach me how to live. Who knew I would find my personal rule book on skid row? Wow.

I made it from the park bench to the amazing life I have today by doing what I have outlined in this book. On the park bench, I could no longer comprehend what words meant. I was angry 24/7 and I was violent on a daily basis. Basically, I was an animal. Today, I am working on my second master's degree, have wonderful friends and I have written this book. Life is so good. If I could tell you only one thing that would change your life—only one thing—it would be to alter your perspective and your attitude (okay, that's two things). When I moved from believing nothing was my fault to knowing I was completely responsible for my life, everything changed. Everything!

Well, at least it seemed as if everything (and even everyone) changed. But is that really what happened?

Actually, it was me that changed. I moved to a different part of my circle. I moved from the dark side of myself to the light side of myself—all within me—without losing me. I see my whole self as a complete circle, containing my persona, my brain, my body, everything that makes up me. Many changes occur within that circle but the circle itself does not change.

This book is about my journey from darkness into light. Throughout our lives we all have negative and positive aspects and traits. I formerly lived mostly within the negative aspect of me. Today, my personality projects my positive side. Many people have shared concerns like, "If I change, I won't be me and maybe I won't like being someone else." This change is not about becoming someone else; this change is about becoming your authentic self—becoming who you were born to be. Genuine, positive change is moving from the dark side of your circle to the light side.

Carol Davis

Waiting

There is a light flickering within me
Waiting to grow and glow.
There is a symphony within me
Waiting to be played.
There is a song with me
Waiting to be sung.
There is a book within me
Waiting to be read.

Oh, Great Spirit, open the door to my heart and soul.
Release the truth within me
Waiting to be felt
To be heard
To be seen.

Changeless Change

Changeless Change

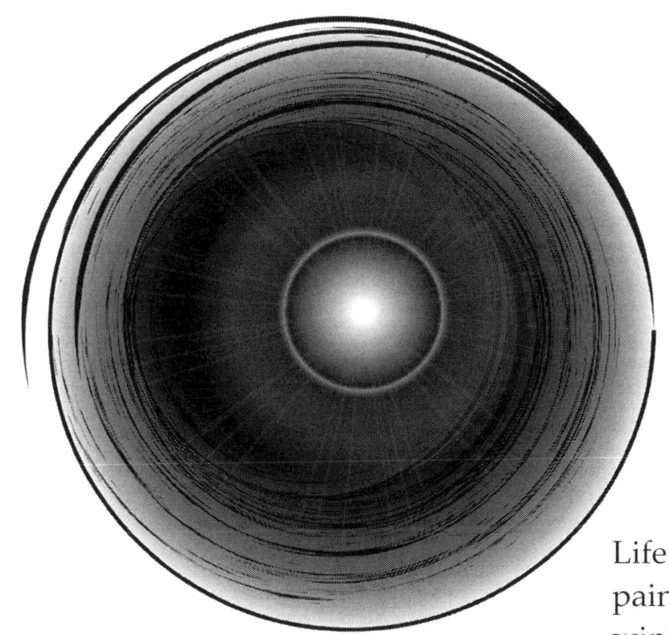

Life is a circle. We are born, we feel joy, we feel pain, we die—that is a full circle of life. Fall, winter, spring and summer, year after year after year for eternity, seasons change within the circle. Each season may differ from year to year, yet the order of the seasons never changes, hence, Changeless Change.

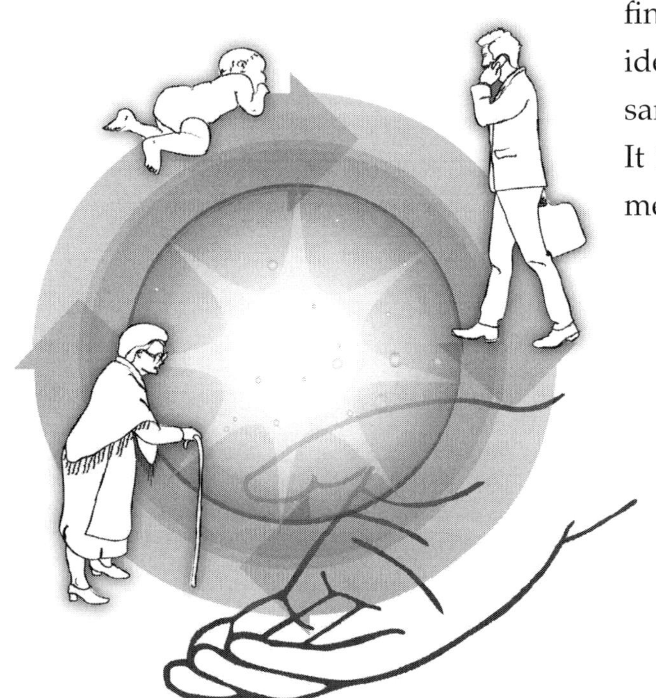

All of life is a series of circles within the big Life Circle. I like circles because understanding them helps me identify my growth and helps me heal. Even when working with another person, whether a professional or a friend, I sometimes find it difficult to see change within myself. But identifying my changes when my life feels the same day after day helps build my self-esteem. It is important to be able to say, "Hey, look at me—I Am changing."

Circle of Pain

We each have our own personal circle made up of our personality, how we function, what we believe, how we act and react. In what I call my Circle of Pain, I can see the process I go through to get away from hurting. Without the symbol of the circle, I too easily think I am running the same old patterns.

However, with the circle image I can clearly see I don't stay in the negative phases as long as I once did and I do stay in positive phases longer. I literally draw this pattern out in a circle so I can see the change within the Changeless Change.

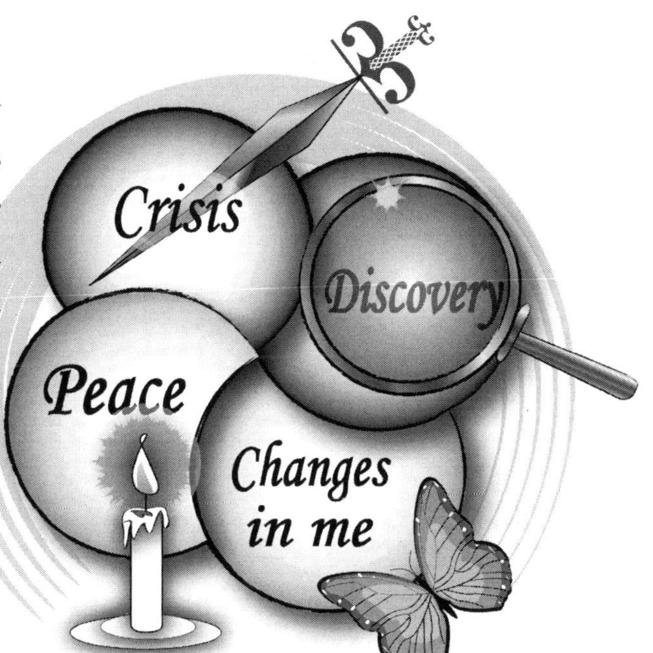

Circle of Seasons

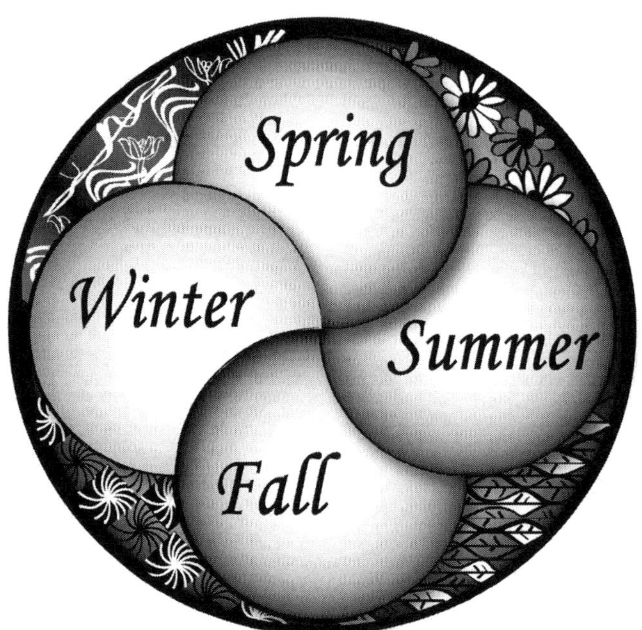

The ever-constant order of the seasons that still allows for change shows us there are lessons to be learned by observing nature.

Is a tree that has let go of its leaves in the autumn of life, or the one standing barren in the winter of life, any less of a tree than the one in full bloom in the spring of life, or the one offering shade and a cool respite in the summer of life?

Nature

On my journey from darkness to light, the first place I began to see hope was in nature. When closely observing patterns in nature I could plainly see answers to challenges and obstacles in my life.

Answers to my problems in nature? Are you kidding me?

Seriously, I really do love studying nature for clarity when I have questions about life; questions like, which way is really correct? There are as many answers as there are people, it seems—different cultures, many colors, people unlike me. How come they…? Why can't they…? Which way is correct?

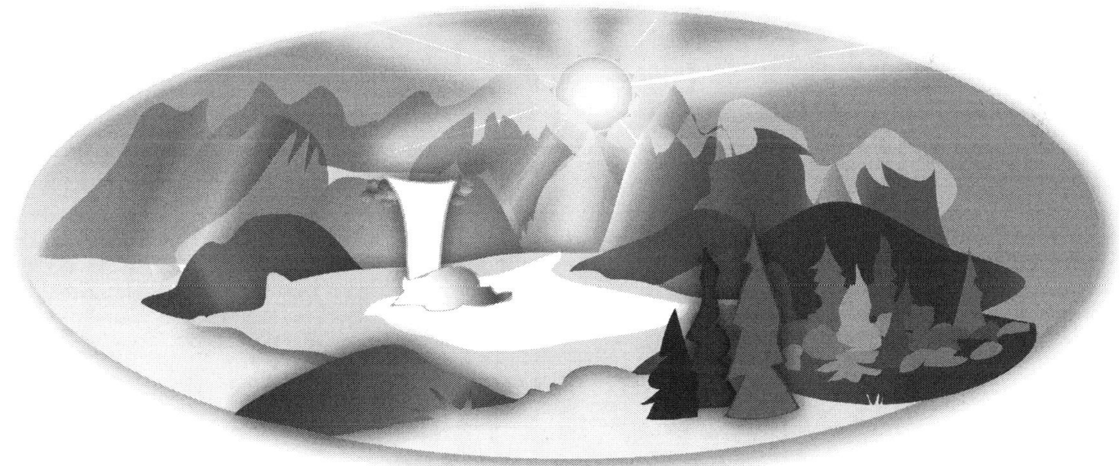

In nature there is no right, no wrong, just differences. When I observe nature, I see why diversity is so significant. There is no one way to do, or believe, or just be.

Judgment in nature is unwarranted.

I was sitting on my porch one day watching a mulberry tree lose its leaves. When I looked around I saw another tree that was keeping its leaves. We never ask the questions of nature that we ask of each other. No one is going to judge a mulberry tree for losing its leaves while another tree keeps its leaves. And what about the multi-colored leaves falling from a variety of trees in autumn? Granted, some people have favorite colors but do they become judgmental about leaves of different colors?

I soon realized how boring the forest would be if all trees were the same. Diversity brings such beauty to the canvas. Like the trees, we all have a place and a purpose. We all have a place where we stand tall and express like no other.

Even apparent calamities have a specific purpose, though we often don't see this during times of trouble. Did you know it takes only 30 seconds for a hailstorm to completely destroy a crop a farmer has nurtured all season? The hail doesn't care if it is two days away from harvest. A hailstorm isn't personal; it is nature at work.

Relationships often feel like hailstorms. Being in nature can remind us that relationships also have their cycles within circles. Speaking of nature and relationships, did you know people are like turnips? Some people love them, some people hate them, but there is nothing wrong with the turnip.

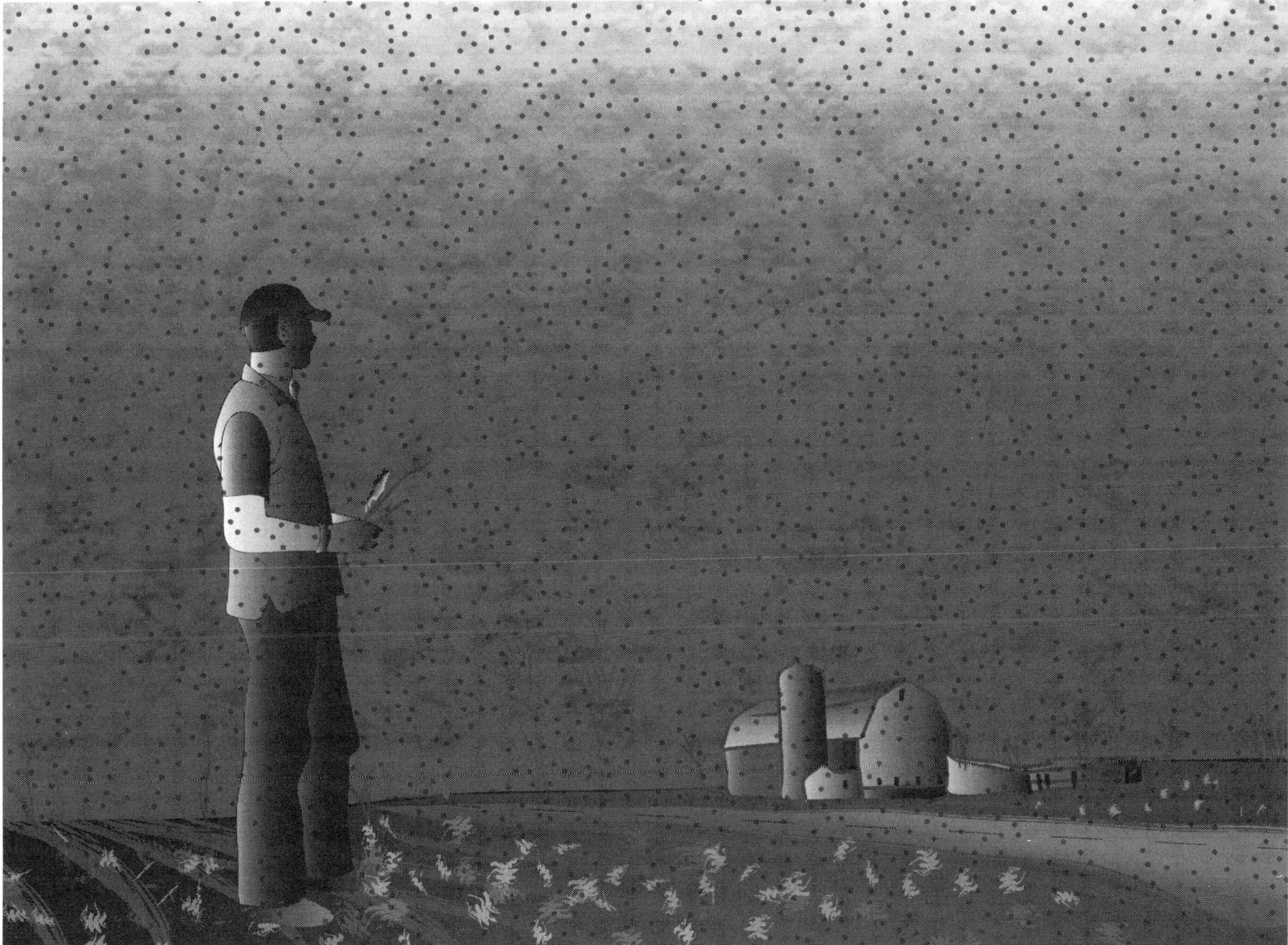

Planting Seeds
(or New Ideas)

I planted my first flower garden from seeds. Wow, what a project that was. Every day I went to my garden and stared at it, wondering how long it would be before a flower popped up. I watered my seeds and I fed them and I waited.

After a few weeks, still nothing. I wanted to dig up the dirt to see if something was happening under the surface. But, I continued to wait and one day when I was not looking, flowers started to break through the soil.

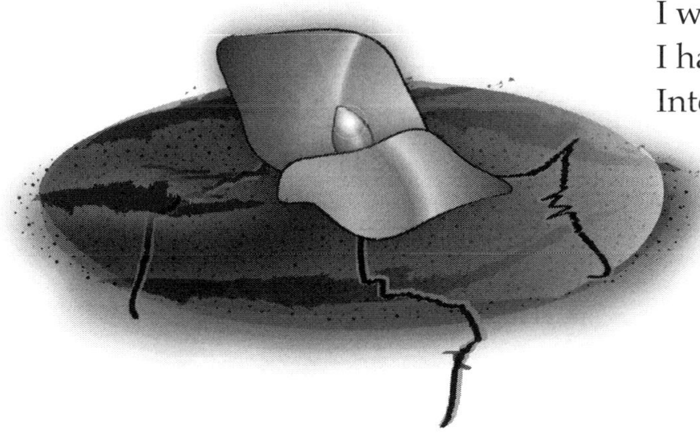

I was so happy, and at that very moment I knew I had learned to trust—to trust the process of an Intelligence greater than me that expresses Itself in me and in you and in those little seeds. How could each seed know what it should grow up to be if that were not the case?

When we "plant" ideas into the universe, it often takes time for our thoughts to bloom or to manifest our visions. That does not mean nothing is happening.

Sometimes when we plant seeds, it looks like dirt for a long time.

No worries; the dirt is also part of the circle.

Once my seeds grew into beautiful, recognizable flowers, the weeds somehow, without my permission, also appeared. Another lesson.

Pull the Weeds

While They Are Still Small

Tending to our gardens includes pulling up the weeds at the root while they are still small enough to easily handle.

Initially, pulling new weeds is actually more about trying to look good on the surface. But, if we just mow down the weeds when we mow the lawn, what usually happens? Underneath the surface, the weeds are spreading like fire. They are spreading, and getting thicker and stronger. Wow. All too soon there is a serious problem and tons more work to do because the weeds have overgrown the lawn. No more faking it now. No more looking good on the surface—the jig is up!

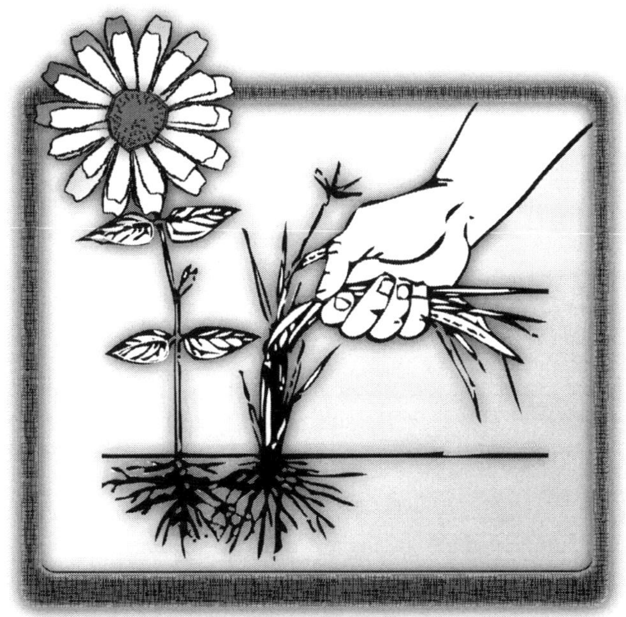

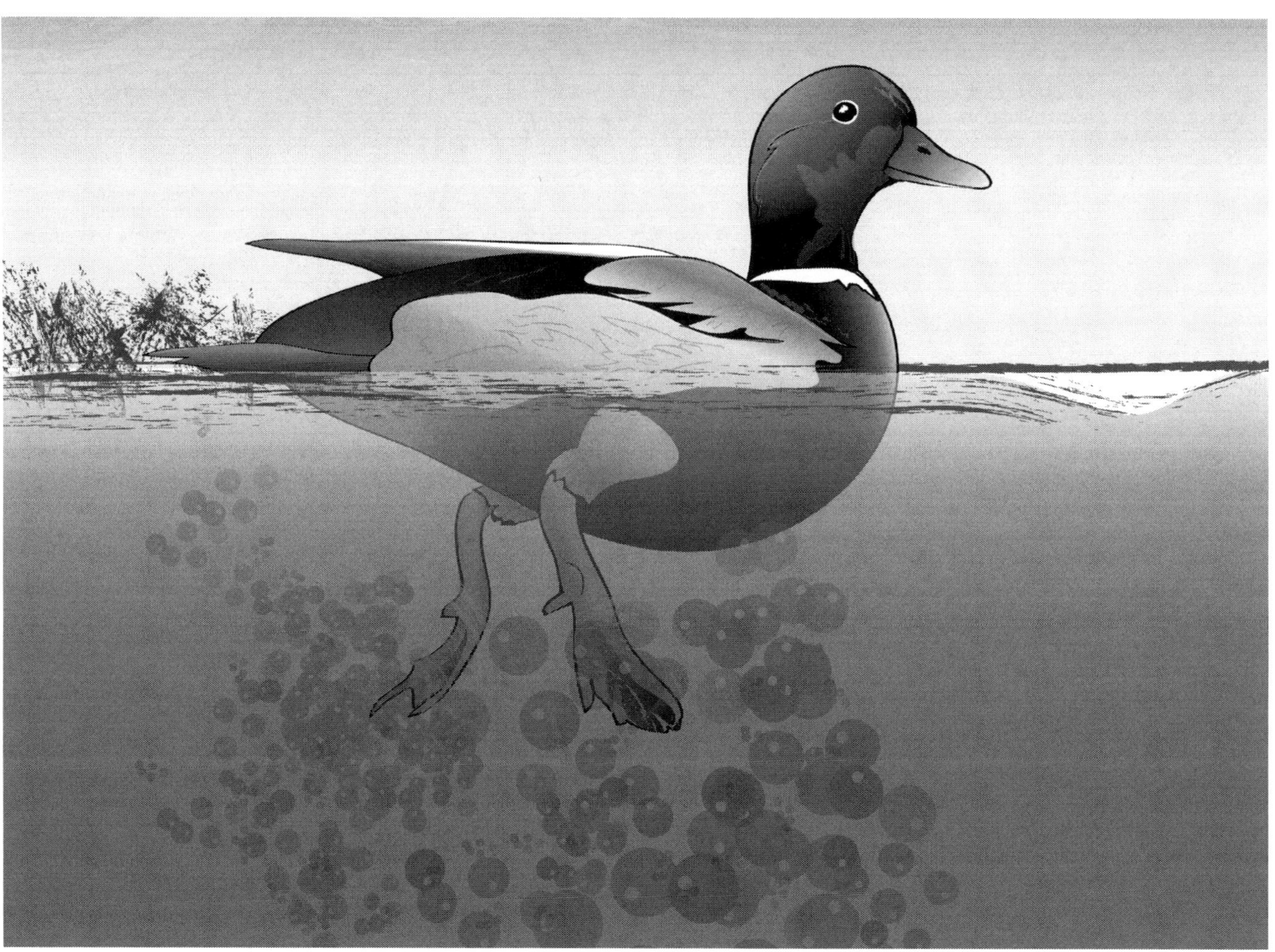

Speaking of Looking Good on the Surface...

I love watching ducks glide across the water. It appears to be so effortless but we do not see below the surface where their little webbed feet are paddling like crazy.

How about you? Do you look calm, serene, and all together on the outside? Underneath the surface are you paddling like crazy? Too many of us are simply trying to stay afloat and look good.

Other folks really are at peace because they have worked hard beneath the surface—weeding, searching, unpacking, evaluating, trashing.

So, don't wait to do your weeding. You delay—you pay.

Tend to the garden that is you, daily. Dig up and discard the "weeds" of your being—every day. It is not only easier to keep up with the task daily, but you might also save money on trips to doctors and pharmacies. This is the circle of your life.

While daily maintenance keeps your weeds from rooting too deeply, there is also a time and a season to not take further action, to be still, to wait, to just be. Sometimes when "bad" things happen that confuse us, it is beneficial to be still before jumping into action again.

It really is your choice. You choose your actions and reactions to life. Your attitude and perceptions are your choice.

Really? Is it always my choice? What about when especially bad things happen?

Actually, I choose my reactions and actions no matter the circumstance. Sometimes I need only change my attitude. Sometimes I need to take action.

And sometimes I simply need to wait.

Wait?

Wait

Just Be

Yes. Wait.

Once again, an answer can be found in nature. The sun is always shining. We sometimes need to wait for the clouds or the storm to pass, but eventually we do see the ever patient and constant sun and often, a delicious rainbow gift as well.

Just Be
Just Be
Just be in this moment

Just Know
Just know in this moment

Just be.... just know....

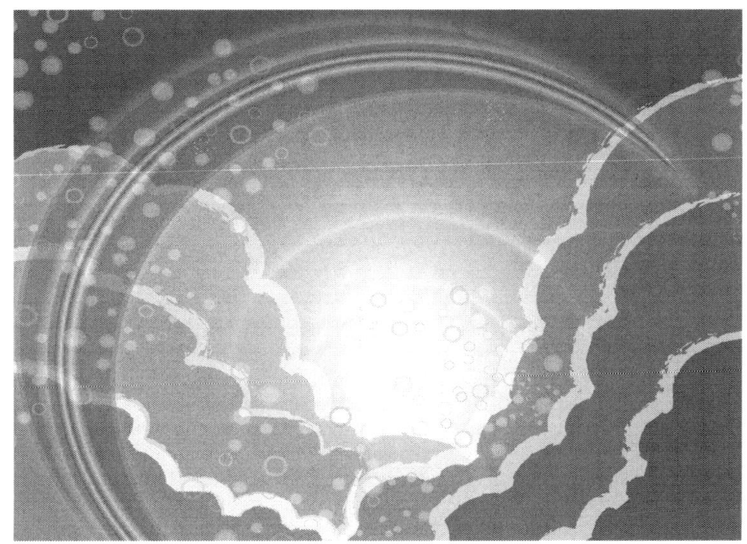

In this moment

All the love, joy, beauty, power, and light in the universe is in you

In this moment

Just Be.

After observing nature for a good while, I started thinking about how all the beauty and precision of nature came about. Of course, that precipitated much study and conversation about the power behind the creation of this amazing planet and this thing called life.

I became quite obsessed with finding just the right, or correct, Higher Power.

"Oh, my gosh," I said to one of my teachers. "So many ways to do everything. Which way is the right way?"

The right way?

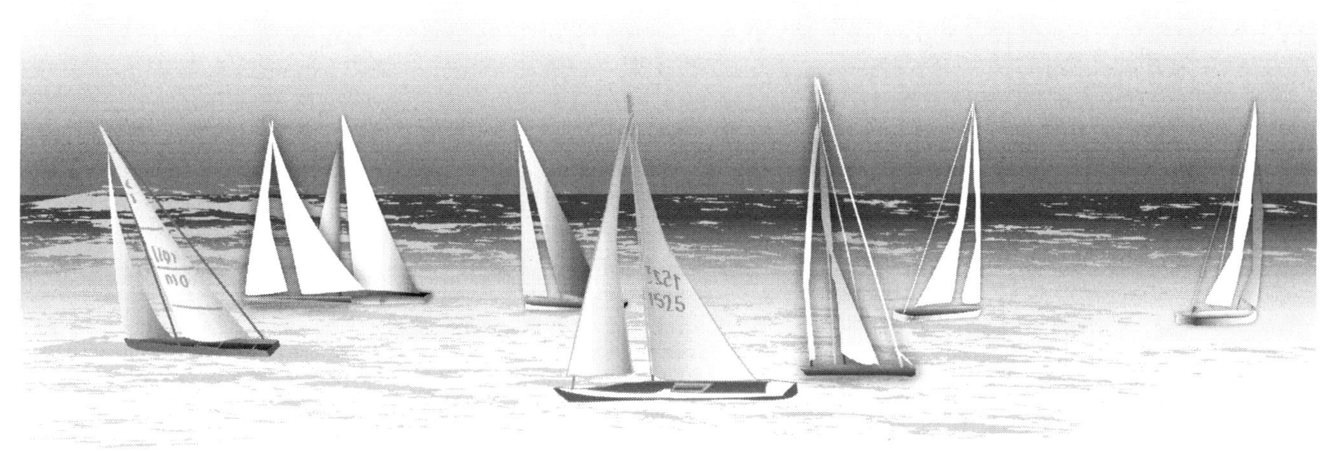

Only One Wind

One day my teacher walked me to his big bay window overlooking the ocean. He said to me, "See those sailboats out there? They are all going in different directions yet there is only one wind, and they are all using the same wind. The direction they sail is contingent upon how they tend their sails."

No path is better or worse than any other path so there is no need to judge or to criticize.

What direction are you sailing?

I finally discovered that the direction I sailed was not as important as knowing there is a Supreme Source, a Creator behind all I see—my Higher Power.

How to access this Power became my newest dilemma. I was confused for a long time about where to find It and how to use It. My selfish, self-centered self could not figure out how It worked.

I often asked my teacher, "Why isn't this Power showing up for me? Where is my good?" (Obviously, I needed to learn how to recognize "good," but that's for another story).

Then, Ta-da! I realized if It was small enough for me to figure out, It would not be big enough to run the universe, or able enough to help you and me at the same time.

One day a picture of a water faucet popped into my head and I grasped, at that very moment, the answer. It is all up to me.

The Source of my good is always present, always available to me. My Source has many names: God, Spirit, Buddha, Allah, Higher Power, and countless more. What the Power is called is not as significant as what It does—and even more importantly, what you believe It does.

But even when I came to understand that the Power, not I, would make a tree I planted rise to the sky, or a flower grace my garden with its blooms, even then I could not believe that same Energy or Creative Power had any interest in me.

Turn on the Faucet

One day I suddenly "got" that my access to the Power was totally up to me. It was always there, waiting for me to say yes.

There is absolutely a Power greater than me. It is in me, always read to express Itself through me, and as me.

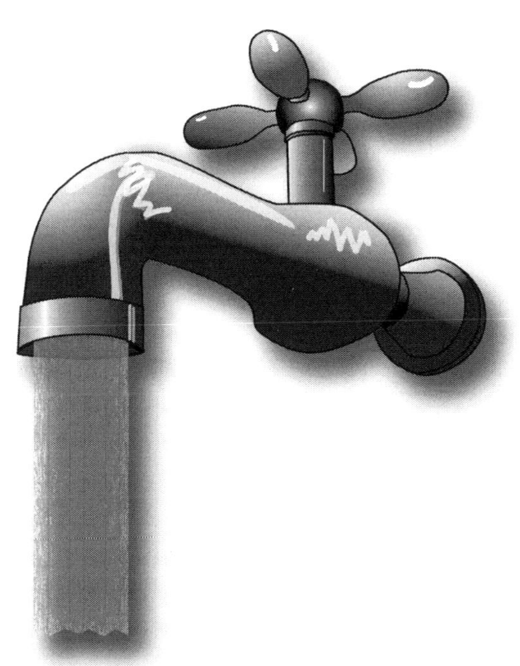

It is up to me to turn that faucet on and allow my good to flow, or to let it drip, or to shut it down.

Always, my choice—good, or not so good.

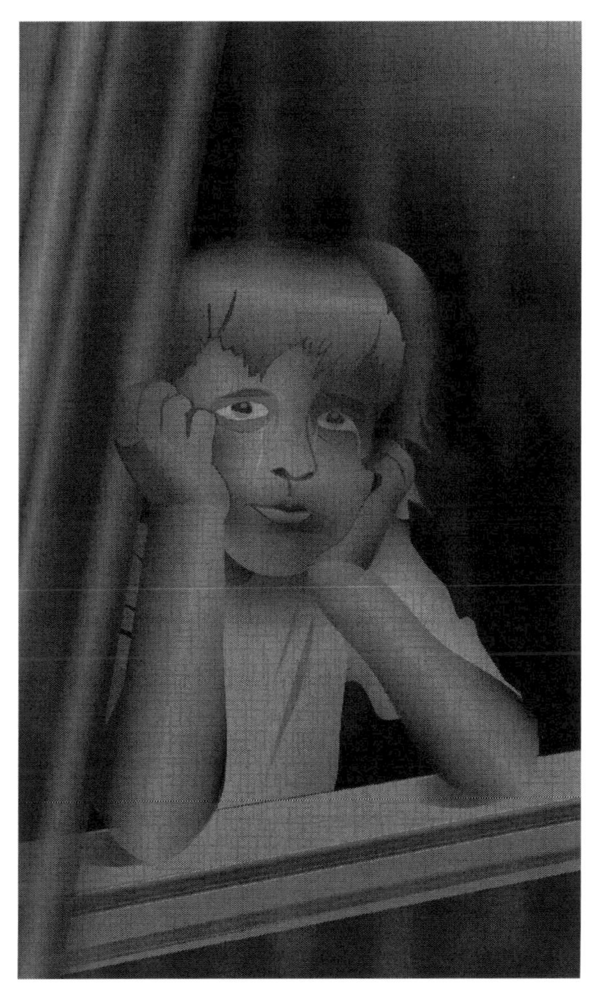

But It Is Not My Fault!!!

Why should I have to work on myself when I did nothing wrong? How come "they" don't have to do anything? People are mean to me and I have to work on my reaction?

Actually, you do not have to do anything, unless you want to feel better; feel some peace and calm and feel good about who you are. Otherwise, stay angry. You are always at choice.

The problem is not what is happening to me, or what "they" are saying to me, or even about me.

The problem—or the solution—stems from how I react.

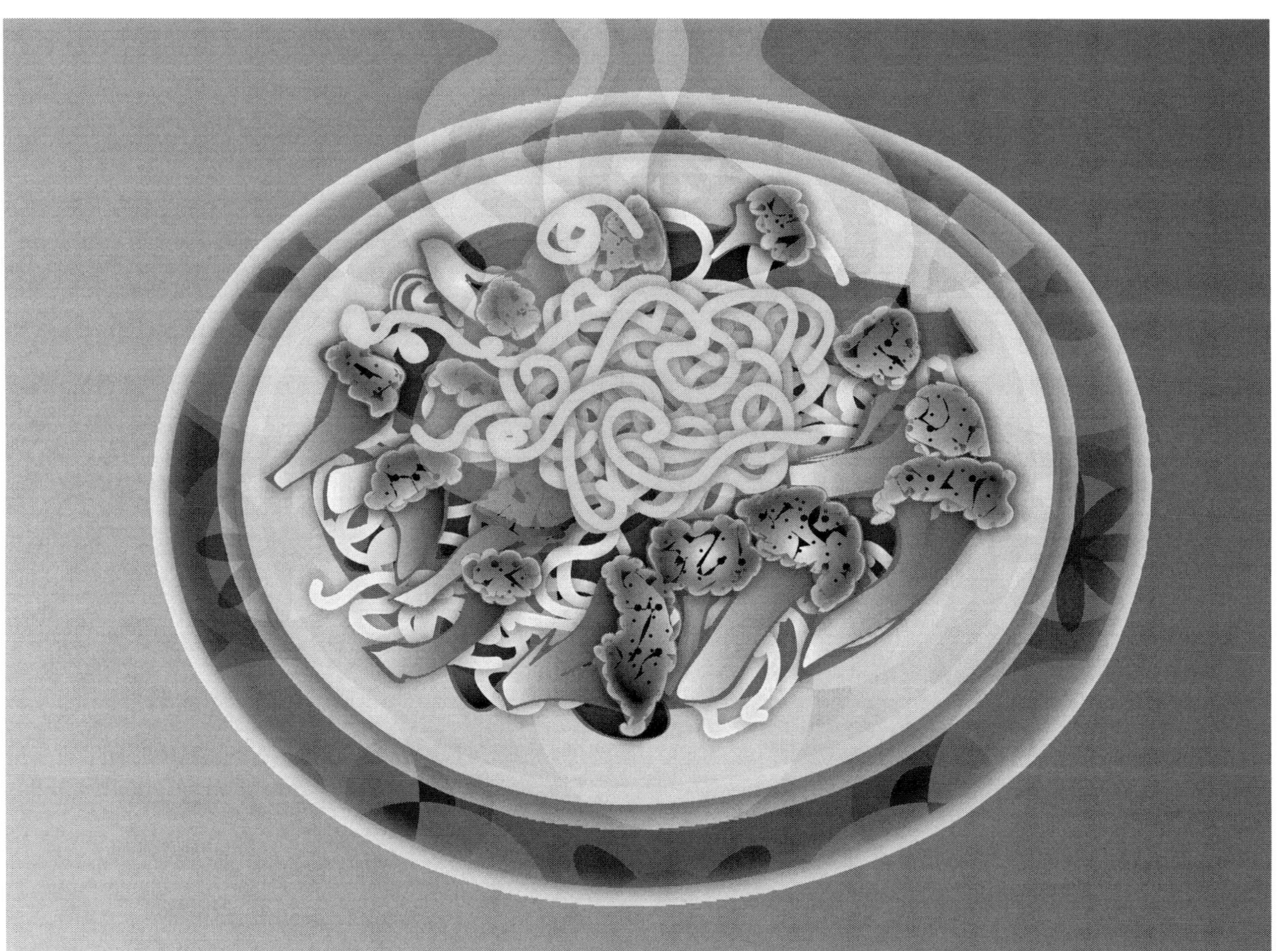

Now for the Main Course!

Yum, yum. Let the work begin!

Now that I have given you an overview of the menu, the time has come to put it all together and start cooking up solutions. Today is a new day. Which recipes will you choose?

Today is a special day.

It is one of a kind.

This day has never been before.

This day will never be again.

It is a new dawn; a new day,

So I greet this day in a whole new way.

Never before have I been here,

So I give it a "Hey!" I give it a cheer!

I will never see this day again,

So let it begin.

I will live this day

As if I'm with a special person

I will never see again.

My eyes are open wide; I will not hide

From the gifts, the joys, the lessons,

Or, the ride.

What a glorious ride, with God as my Guide.

Releasing the Agony of Imperfection

How do you feel when you make a mistake?

I hate making mistakes! We all know everyone makes mistakes and many people seem to accept that and move on. For others, making a mistake is so painful that the inner storm of discontent is only quieted by the abuse of alcohol, or drugs, or food, or by doing violence to the self or others.

Why, the question is asked. Why??? The slightest mistake—inadvertently hurting someone's feelings, or forgetting a document for a meeting—can trigger the "Agony of Imperfection." I do not know why. I do know the source for me and I recommend finding out when you learned the lie that it is not okay to make mistakes. For me, it was the belt. If I made the slightest mistake, any mistake, my father beat my body with a belt. So now, I know the shame that overwhelms me when I make a mistake is me waiting for the belt. After I left home, I beat myself. But now I know better; today there is no more belt.

Go back in time and listen for the person who said to you, "Shame on you!" Who is that? Who is saying that to you? Identify that person and know they told you a lie.

It is okay to be wrong. It is okay to make a mistake. It is okay to "fail." Let go of the belt.

Write a New Life Story.

You are amazing and you have many more important things to do than to worry about being perfect. Perfectionism is so very painful.

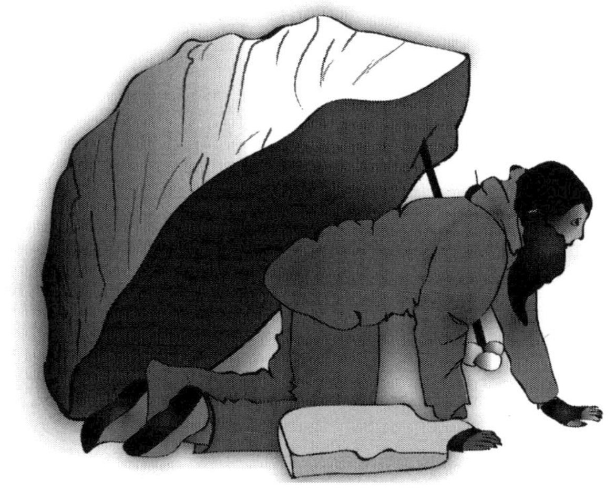

Today, I no longer use substances of any kind to quiet the storm. Today, I look within and see when I learned the lies. Then, when I feel the agony or have a "shame attack," I call someone, talk it out, and I shrink it!

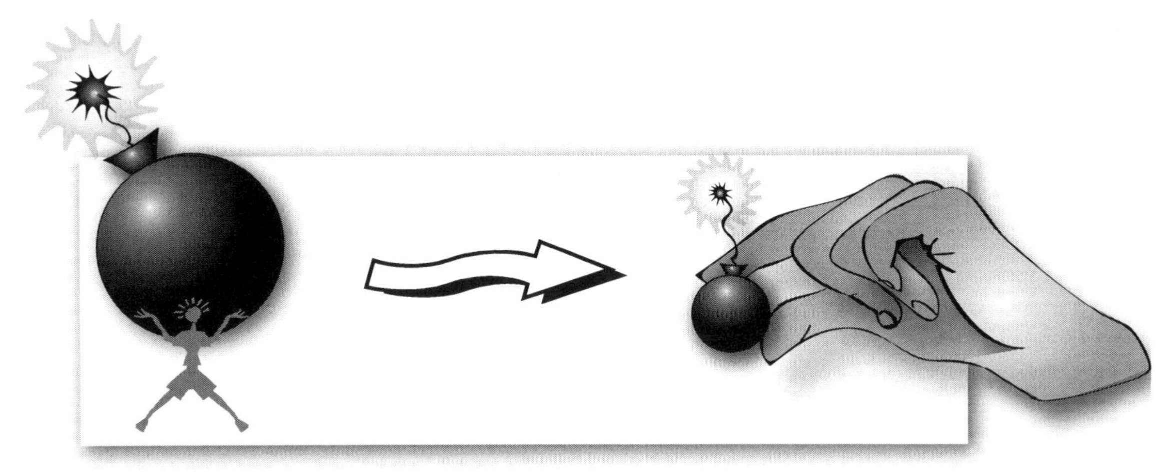

Shrink It

Shrink it? Shrink what? Shrink anything, or anyone bothering you. When I feel hurt or intimidated by people I shrink them into little children and they are way less scary.

You can also try the shrinking technique with any of your emotions. The next time you are overwhelmed with debilitating shame, squeeze that emotion into a small ball and put it in a box until you are ready to deal with it.

Scales of Justice

One night many years ago, I sat straight up in bed with a vision of the "scales of justice." I had been harboring resentment (re-feeling over and over) for months about the behavior of a particular person.

Of course, I saw myself as the "good" person and him as the "bad" person. If that is true, I thought while picturing the scales, then how come I am wide awake and the "bad guy" is probably sleeping like a rock? The vision of the scales helped me put my perception and attitude back in balance by reminding me that I choose my reactions. I made a choice in that moment not to torture myself, and never again have I lost sleep due to resentment. I just picture those scales and I am okay.

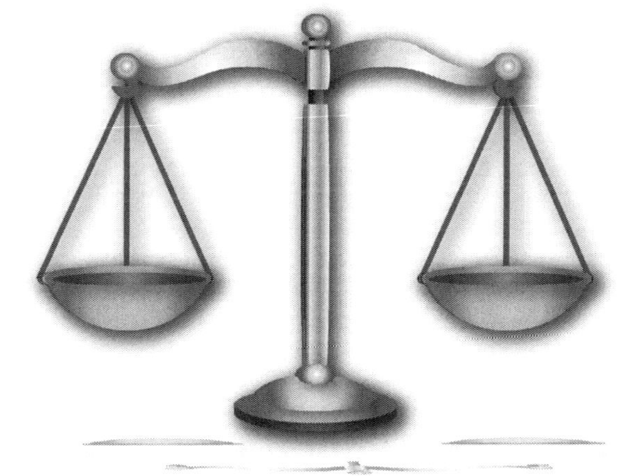

Well, I'm okay as far as sleeping is concerned. But I realized I needed to begin work on a lifetime of resentments and I did this by taking inventory in "the attic" of my life, where my past is stored. However, before I could get there I needed to address my anger and rage.

But how?

I was way too angry to write. My teachers said, "Just start writing anyway—just one page. Write down the name of someone." But, I could not do that. I would start raging at just the thought of someone in my past. I was no longer acting out violently against people or property that was not mine, but I raged and smashed things—my own things. Crazy.

People kept telling me I needed to "deal with my anger" and that made me angry. I yelled, I was mean and hurtful. What to do?

When I was angry I felt like a balloon filled to the brim with air had been let go inside of me. Have you ever seen that… a balloon releasing air, flying every which way in a room like a psycho bird? That is how I felt inside when I was that angry—like balls were bouncing in every direction, uncontrollably, inside of me.

A Good Beating

One day I got the wild idea to beat up my bed. Yes, every time I felt the rage I would pummel my bed until the energy inside of me dissipated. Of course, I wasn't always at home so I occasionally had a few "slips of the tongue," but more often I would hold my anger inside, knowing my bed and some sweet release was waiting for me when I did get home.

Releasing the energy of anger within me, I was then able to finally enter into the "attic" of my being to start rummaging through everything buried there.

In my attic I found the clues for beginning my journey back to me.

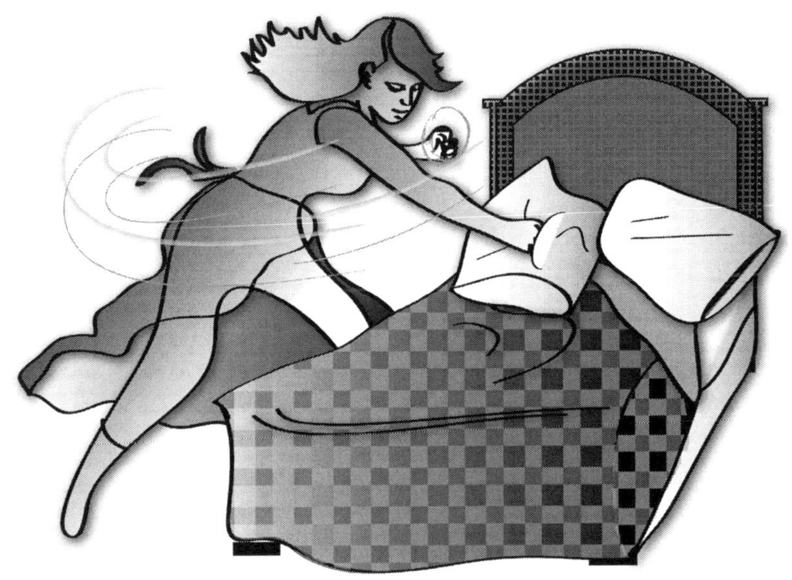

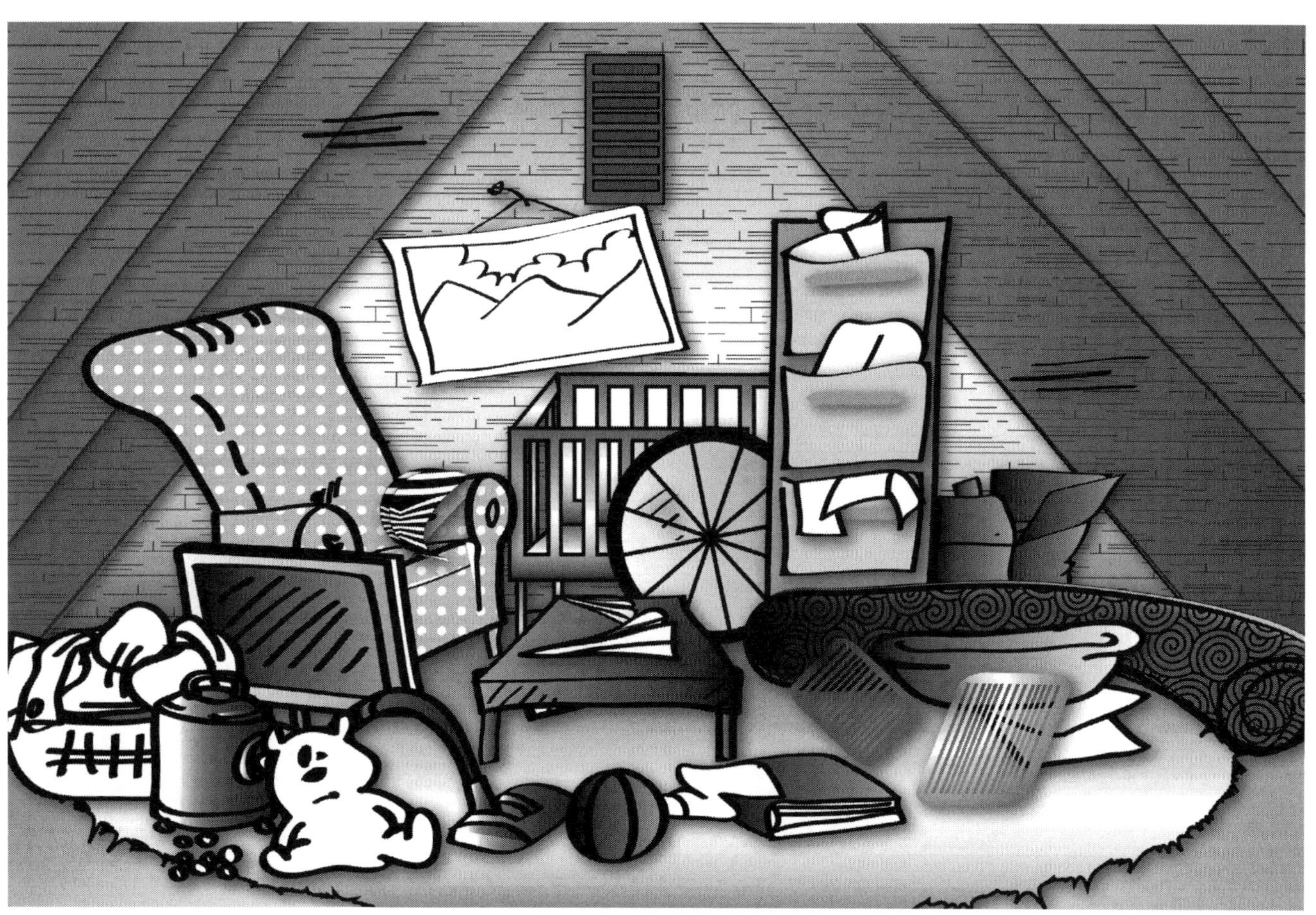

The Attic

All the old ideas I have carried with me since birth are stored in my subconscious mind—the place I call my attic.

Stored in our attics is all we have learned throughout our lives, and mostly what we learned during our first few years on this planet. This is what continues to direct our actions and reactions to everything.

What a powerhouse your attic is! Most of us have no idea that it is the fuel for the engine that spins our minds and directs our actions and reactions.

The information stored in our attics adds instruction and direction every day to what we are reading, or seeing, or being told. Additionally, some of the old stored ideas are added to current any instructions we give. To illustrate this, give someone 15 seconds to completely fill in an outline in a child's coloring book. Chances are they cannot complete the task. Why? Because, their subconscious mind added the instruction from deep within: "Don't color outside the lines."

So, clean out the attic!

This is not a project most of us look forward to. Most of us don't know exactly what is in our attics, or our subconscious minds. Exploring inside can be fun, exhausting, painful, scary, or dismal, and it is definitely not an overnight task. I put it off for a long time—for several years, actually—after I knew I needed to do it. Still, the circles keep turning—changeless change.

Cycles of Life

The amount of time it takes to sort through all that junk stored in the attic depends a bit on where we are in the circle of our lives.

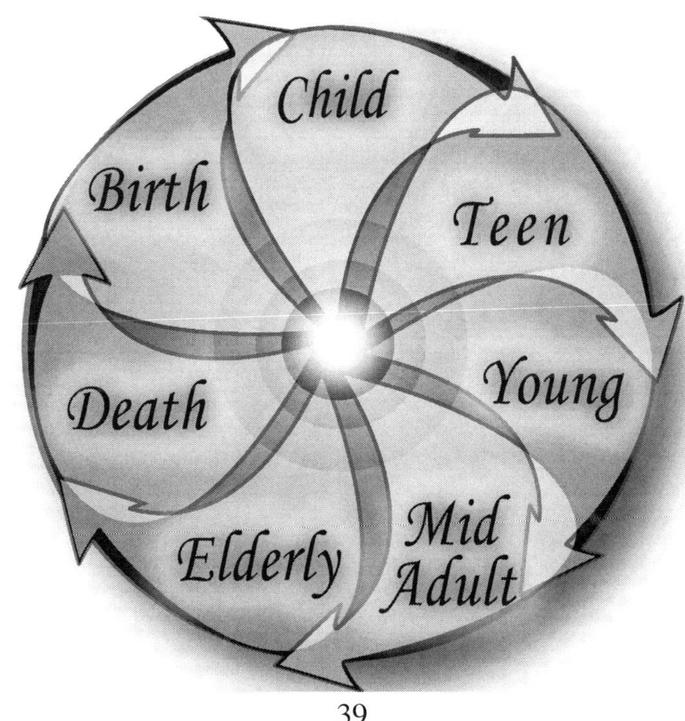

Regardless of our place on the life cycle, we can begin the healing process by writing down the name of the person, place, or thing we first come across in the attic. Chronological order is of no significance.

I want to say a little more about why we need to spend time in the attic. When we are there, we sort through every single thing we see and we carefully delve into each one. We assess each discovery for its value or contribution to our lives and if there is none, we toss it!

There is a very important reason to be on this reconnaissance. A reconnaissance is a mission to obtain information, by visual observation or other detection methods, about the activities and resources of an enemy or potential enemy. And guess what? The enemy, or potential enemy, lives within us. As you may have heard, we are our own worst enemies.

To deal with our baggage, we need to know what is going through the screening.

Baggage screening?

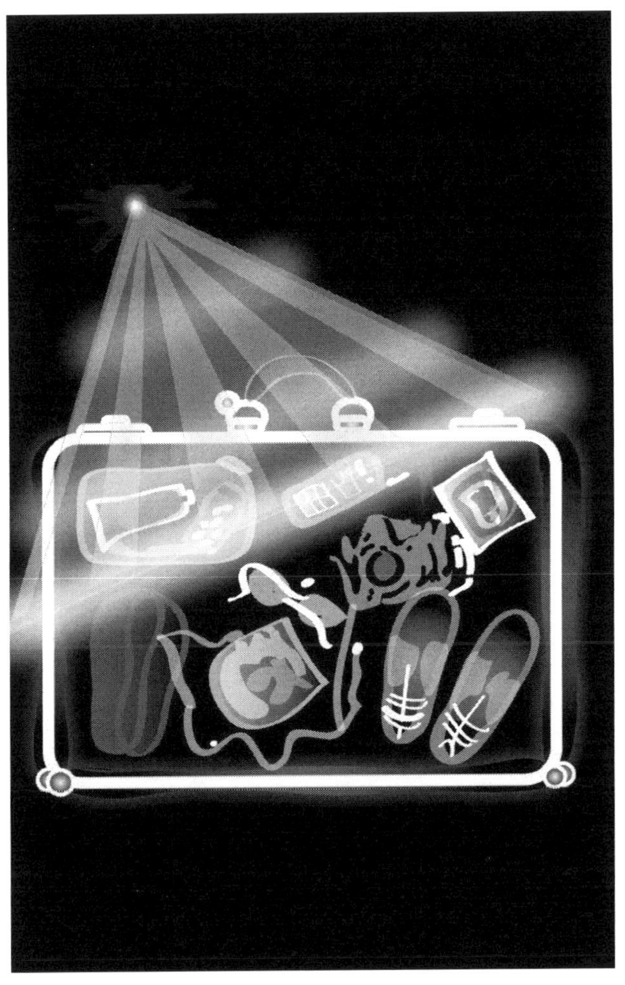

Baggage Screening

The entire process of finding where in the attic information is stored takes place in a nanosecond. The process is not unlike the baggage screening that takes place in airports.

All vehicles of communication…

listening
talking
observing
reading
body language

…go through the x-ray scanners. All the old ideas we have been carrying around, all the instructions and directions we've added to the old ideas, all of it informs our actions and reactions.

Now that we know why we must look at our baggage, let's talk about how we clean out the attic.

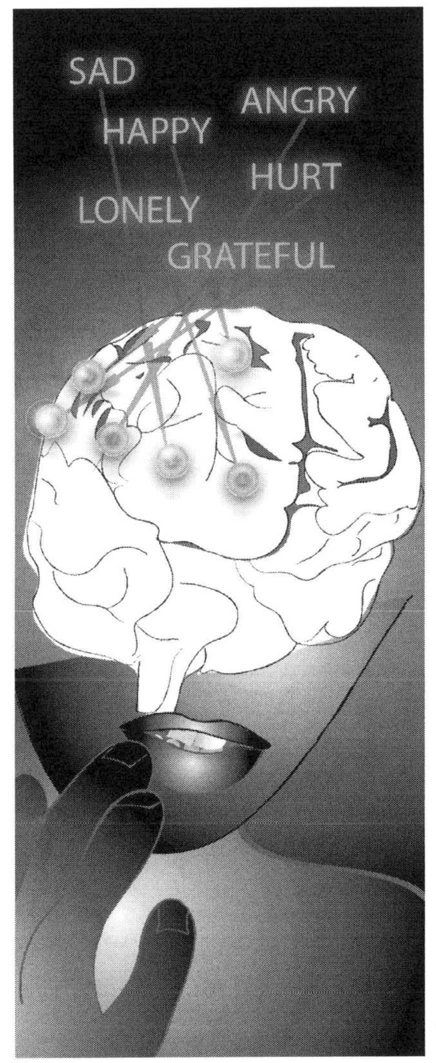

Rooms for Rent

Seeing "rooms" in my attic helps me get in touch with why I am feeling certain feelings. For example: I was watching a movie that had nothing to do with death or sickness, but all of a sudden, I became sad and started crying because I missed my deceased sister.

I thought, What the heck is that about? Apparently, something sad did happen in the movie that took me into the sad room. Once in that room, I was in touch with all the sad memories stored there.

The rooms in my attic do not differentiate between minor and major events. This can be problematic, especially in the angry room. Have you ever felt intense anger, or even rage, for no apparent reason? Everything seems okay in your life, nothing major going on, but suddenly you are lashing out at someone?

For me, the smallest annoyance would take me to the angry room, and there, I was exposed to all the perceived wrongs done to me since forever! Having this knowledge of stored past issues helped me move into and deal with the reality of the present, and most often my anger, once acknowledged, subsided.

Sometimes, however, I needed to do some writing to find out where the feeling was coming from. Whenever I write about my feelings I discover something new about me that helps me be a better person.

The Magic Trick

Taking Inventory

Taking my own inventory in writing—on paper—is a very magical tool. Yes, Magic!

Writing is like magic. Take out a piece of paper and a pen or pencil and write the old-fashioned way. Tell a story about what you found in the attic. What did it look like? How did it make you feel? Do you want to keep it, or throw it away? This process is very similar to taking inventory in a business—just a little more detailed.

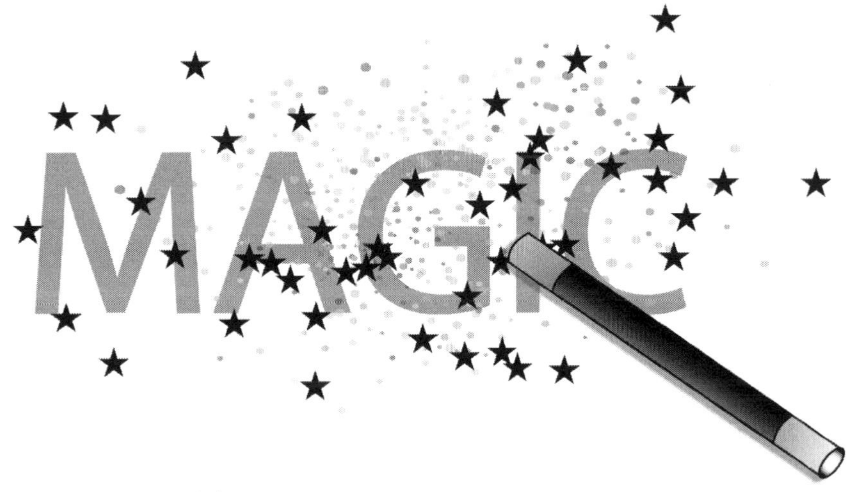

When I write with a pen or pencil on paper (forget technology for now), thoughts appear that were never in my head.

Writing is helpful for many reasons: 1) Identifying my part in a situation; 2) Getting to the true source (the hidden stuff) so I heal faster; 3) Pro and con lists help me make important decisions; and, 4) Just basic house cleaning—getting rid of the old to make room for the new.

Identifying My Part in Any Situation

My life simply does not get any better when I am blaming others or shaming myself. It is my desire to be happy, joyous and free. That does not occur unless I am willing to go through the pain of looking at my part, or am willing to own my reaction to people, places and events. Now, most will say at this point, "Wait just one minute, here. What if someone has committed a crime against me?" As we already know, there are many times when we believe we are not at fault.

"It's Not My Fault!" is the most common reason to stay sad or angry and not look at your own reactions—your part in any predicament. This house cleaning is not about being right or wrong. It is about you getting comfortable with you. It is about not being a doormat. It is about living in a state of peace and joy, regardless of what "they" are doing to you. It is not about the situation at all. It is about you and your reactions. You say, "Anyone would be angry" in certain situations. Maybe yes. Maybe no.

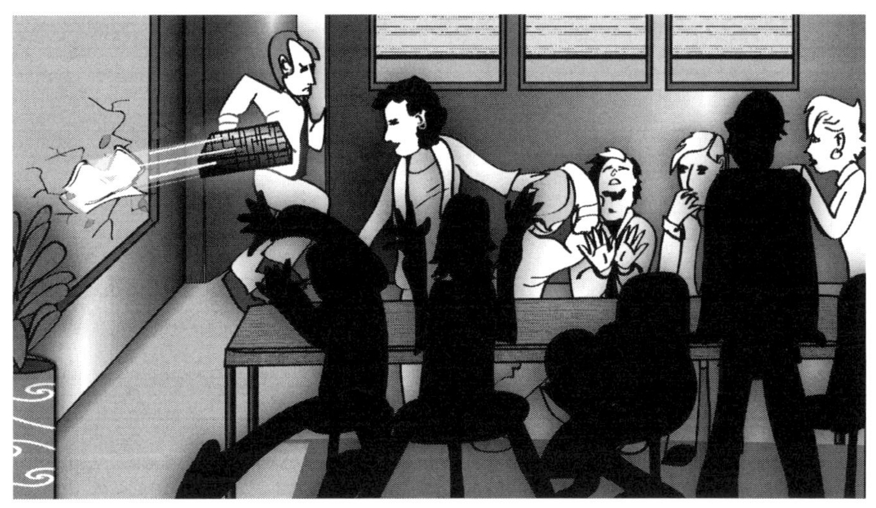

Ten people are sitting in a room having a discussion. This room has a large bay window and out of the clear blue, a brick suddenly smashes through the window. For the purpose of this illustration, let's agree this is a criminal act of violence against ten innocent people. In spite of there being 100% agreement on the nature of the event, we could very possibly see 10 different reactions. How can that be? It happens because our reactions are a result of the baggage we drag around, and everyone's baggage is different. Remember, everything we see, hear, touch, feel, and experience first goes through the baggage scanner and gives us instructions about how to react.

One person may have a reaction similar to the cartoon above. Someone else may feel ill. Yet another might run after the perpetrator. Still another may have the presence of mind to call the police. Others might just sit in a stupor, paralyzed by this horrific act. Bottom line, everyone's reaction will be a result of their own life history—the stuff hidden away in the attic that still directs their lives.

Getting to the True Source

The true source of our discomfort is often attached to a lie we were taught somewhere in the past and often goes back as far as early childhood. That lie has been stored in your attic for a long time and actually adds to any event, real or imagined. Writing about your discomfort makes you feel. If you can uncover when you first felt a certain way you have uncovered a source to be dealt with.

Recall an uncomfortable situation and think about the last time you felt what you are feeling now; and the time before that when you felt the same feeling, and then even before that, and so on. You will uncover patterns that are your very own. You will see how the same stuff keeps happening—the same relationships with different names and different faces, over and over. You can stop the cycle of yourself, for yourself, by yourself, by writing.

When we are done searching the attic and the writing, (for now, as it is a lifetime tool), it is time to "Dump the mud!"

Dump the Mud Out of the Bucket!

Throughout this book I refer to the process of finding where "it" is stored in the attic, evaluating it and then tossing what is not adding to your life. This is a process we must surrender to if we are to be free of any part of the past that blocks us from the sunlight of the life we want.

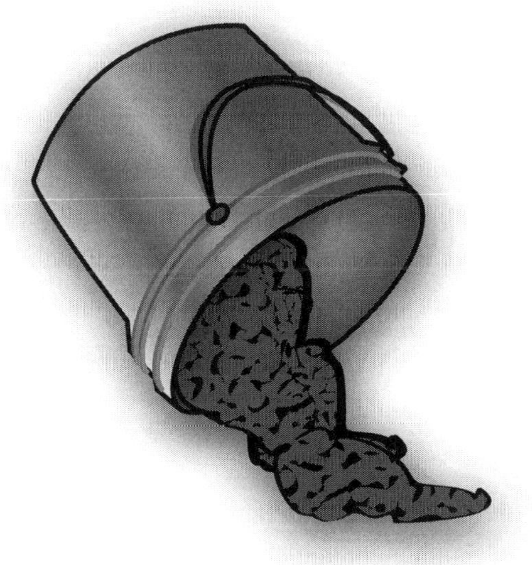

The process is one of taking inventory of ourselves on a regular basis. Sometimes we just think about things, and other times we need to do a thorough written inventory. Part of the inventory process is looking at what we want to keep and what we want to throw away.

Dig it up, haul it out of the attic, and unpack the suitcase.

Look at it. Does it still belong with you?

If it no longer serves you, let it go.

Before I began taking inventory on a regular basis, it was as if I was hauling around a bucket of mud, filled to the brim. I had no room for information about how to live or deal with life until I dumped out the mud and made room for fresh, clean water. (Remember the water faucet?).

Moving On

What Next? Maintenance Steps and Staying Fit!

We need to keep our mental and emotional health fit just as we do our bodies.

Continue regular visits to your attic to take inventory.

Practice forgiveness exercises.

Tend to your marble bag.

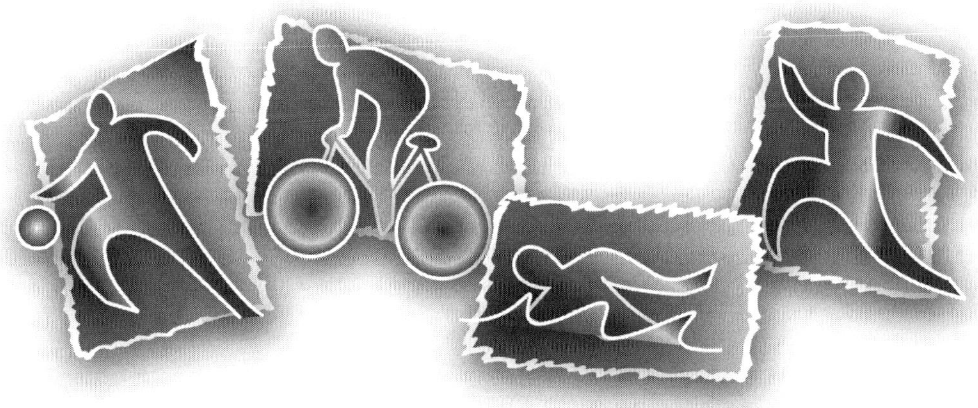

Forgiveness

Here is the short story on forgiveness. It is all about you. Yes, you absolutely have the right to stay angry with someone. You also have the right to stick your finger in a light socket. And the point would be… ???

To forgive is so very awesome. When you forgive, the "bad guy" is no longer in charge and you get to take back your own power!

But how? Every once in a while, I am able to just let go of a person, place, or event when I need to. However, more often it takes work. I try one thing at a time and just keep at it until I just know I am not re-feeling my anger or hurt.

I wish for "them" all the happiness, wellness, and success I would want for myself.

I write out 70 X 7 times: [Name] I forgive you for _______. Yes. 70 times a day for 7 days.

I forgive myself.

Now, what is this marble bag we must tend to?

The Marble Bag

Did you ever wonder why you sometimes "lose it" over the smallest, most insignificant event? It is because your marble bag is full! That happens when we don't deal with issues as they come up because we "don't have time," or "it really isn't that big of a deal."

Think of every irritation you ignore as a little marble. You stuff it away in the marble bag (which is your gut). One day, you try to put another little marble in the bag and it is already overflowing with little marbles (unattended little issues), then Pow! The fireworks explode because there is no more room in the marble bag.

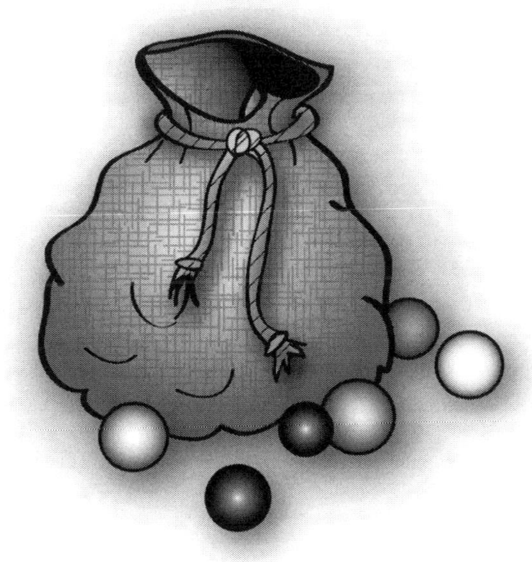

So, stay fit! Keep up the good work you have started.

It is often painful to part with old friends in the attic. I have shed many tears in this process. But those tears are so healing; they are like a shower for your soul. As you do the work of dumping useless stuff out of your attic, you will begin to feel lighter and lighter.

This journey from the darkness into the light is ongoing as you grow and change, but hopefully, you have found or will soon find, as I have, that the reward is greater than the pain.

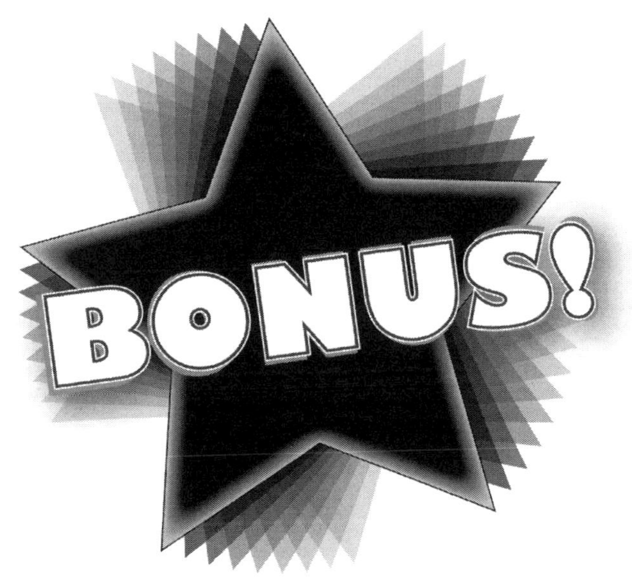

A Few More Thoughts to Ponder

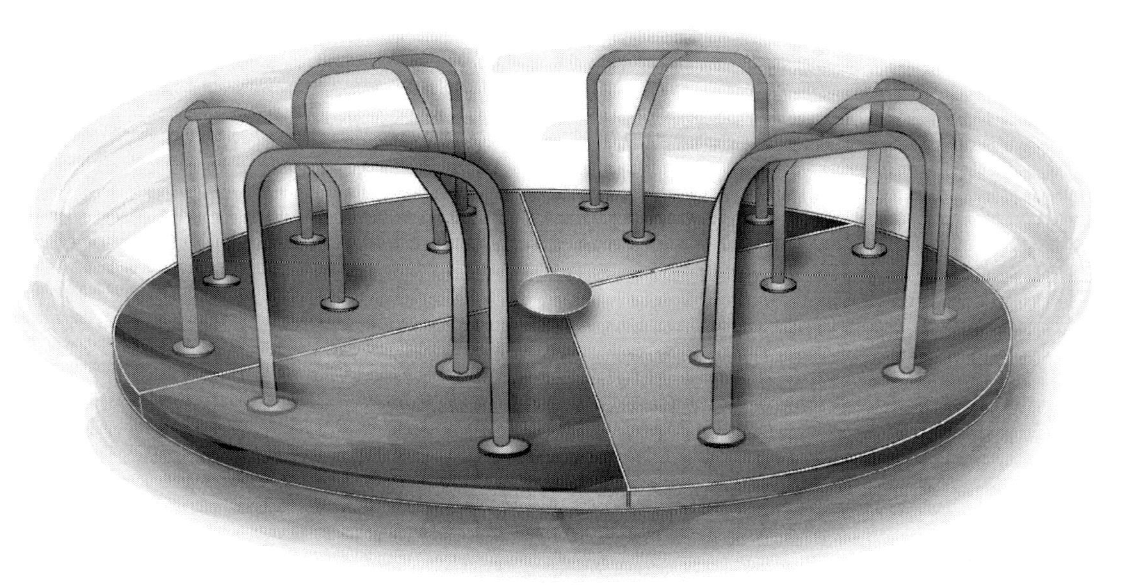

Life Really Is Fair

Yes, we do get what we give. Hence, the age-old adage, "Do unto others as you would have them do unto you."

I know some people do not believe this to be true because it is not clear how it works. I once had a very limited and narrow vision of this. I believed you should give me whatever I gave you; treat me as I treated you. A gives to B, therefore, B should give back to A. It might work that way once in a while, but that is rare.

Picture a spinning Merry-Go-Round. Now visualize throwing something onto it. You have absolutely no idea where it will fly off, but it will. And that is how it works. I never know where or when or how what I put out there (bad as well as good) will come back to me, but it will come back.

A female executive discovers that her husband has been lying to her about some of his activities. She is devastated because she has never lied to him and always believed in the "Golden Rule." However, she often lies to co-workers, subordinates and friends. That is how it works.

We do get what we give—Always.

Communication skills will help you along your way.

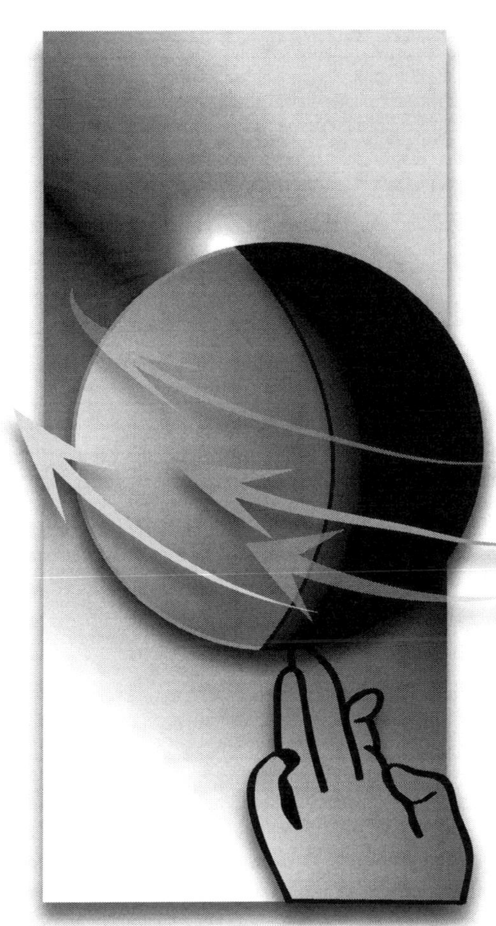

Communication

(C. A. T.)

We often assume another person knows exactly what we mean in our conversations. For example, direct a child to clean his or her room. Unless you clearly define what clean means to you, the end result will be whatever clean means to the child. We also too often assume we know what someone is saying to us.

CLARITY

Clarify the actual words you hear from the person you are communicating with. Define your terms. Do the words you hear mean the same to you as to the one who spoke them? Do not try to be a mind reader, or expect anyone to read your mind.

It's a big mistake to say, "I don't need to clarify anything; I know what I heard." Yes, you may know what you heard, but what does it mean to each of you? There are many examples of not only words but also whole sentences that can be misunderstood. Here is one example: I invite you to visit me. You ask, “How is the weather?” I say, “The weather is perfect!” So, you arrive to visit me and you are madder than heck because it is 95 degrees. You say, “I thought you said it was perfect?” I say, “It is!” Turns out, you are from the beach and perfect to you is 75 degrees. I live in the desert and 95 degrees is perfect for me.

That may be an over simplistic example, but that is how it works.

ATTITUDE

Maintain an attitude of open-mindedness in an argument. No blaming! No shaming! Blaming allows us to stay narrow-minded and to escape from looking at any viewpoint but our own. Blaming is a shaming act and an attempt to make our part be someone else’s fault.

TURN IT AROUND

There is always another side to the story... and then there’s the truth.

Be of Service

Yes, to stay feeling good, volunteer somewhere—hospitals, theaters, libraries, even if only to help out your neighbors. You go to the gym to take care of your body. You read books or work crossword puzzles to take care of your mind. Find a way to help others, every day, to take care of your heart and soul.

Being of service is a win-win situation. When you are helping another, they get what they need; you get a lighter heart and feel good about yourself.

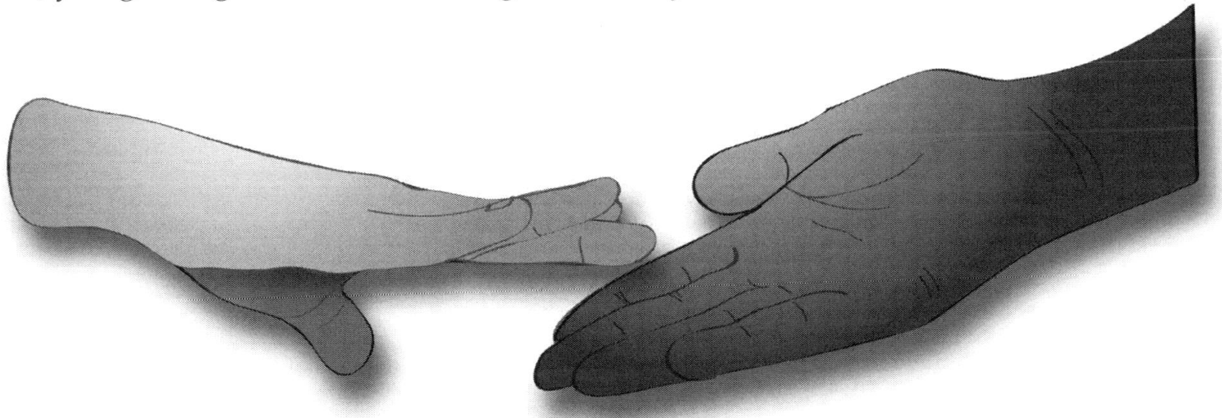

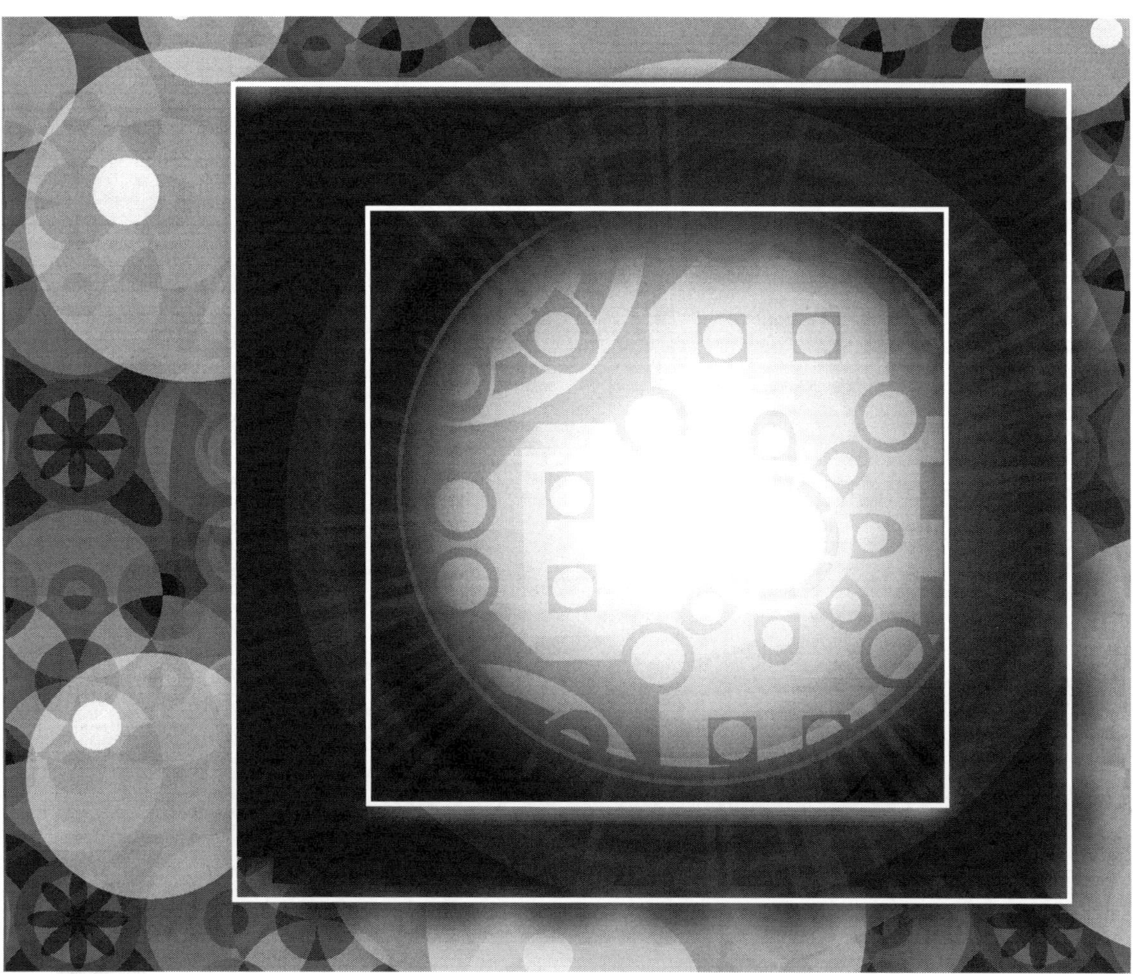

The Circles of Our Lives

Last night at dinner my best friend from high school asked me, "Why have you never married and had children? You always seemed so normal."

I have lived most of my life trying to figure out how to squeeze the big circle of me—the precious, warm, sweet loving being of me—into the little square box of who you want me, or need me, to be. The circle of me is so much more than what you see. It is not what I am doing; it is who I am being. I have dreams, passions, beliefs, ideas, and goals, as most people do, but they may or may not fit into the little box of who I am "supposed to be."

However, my passions and dreams, all I aspire to be, do fit within the circle of my wholeness and the Divine Idea of me. My circle includes the good, the bad, and the ugly—all of me. It is my past, my present, and my future and it does not fit, cannot fit, into your box.

Are you being you? Or are you doing what you believe you are "expected" to do? Sometimes they are the same and that is way cool. However, if there is a fire burning within you to be more and do more, go for it. Jump out of their box and into your circle of your wholeness. Join me in recognizing and accepting the Divine Idea of your beingness. Who are you? What are you here to do?

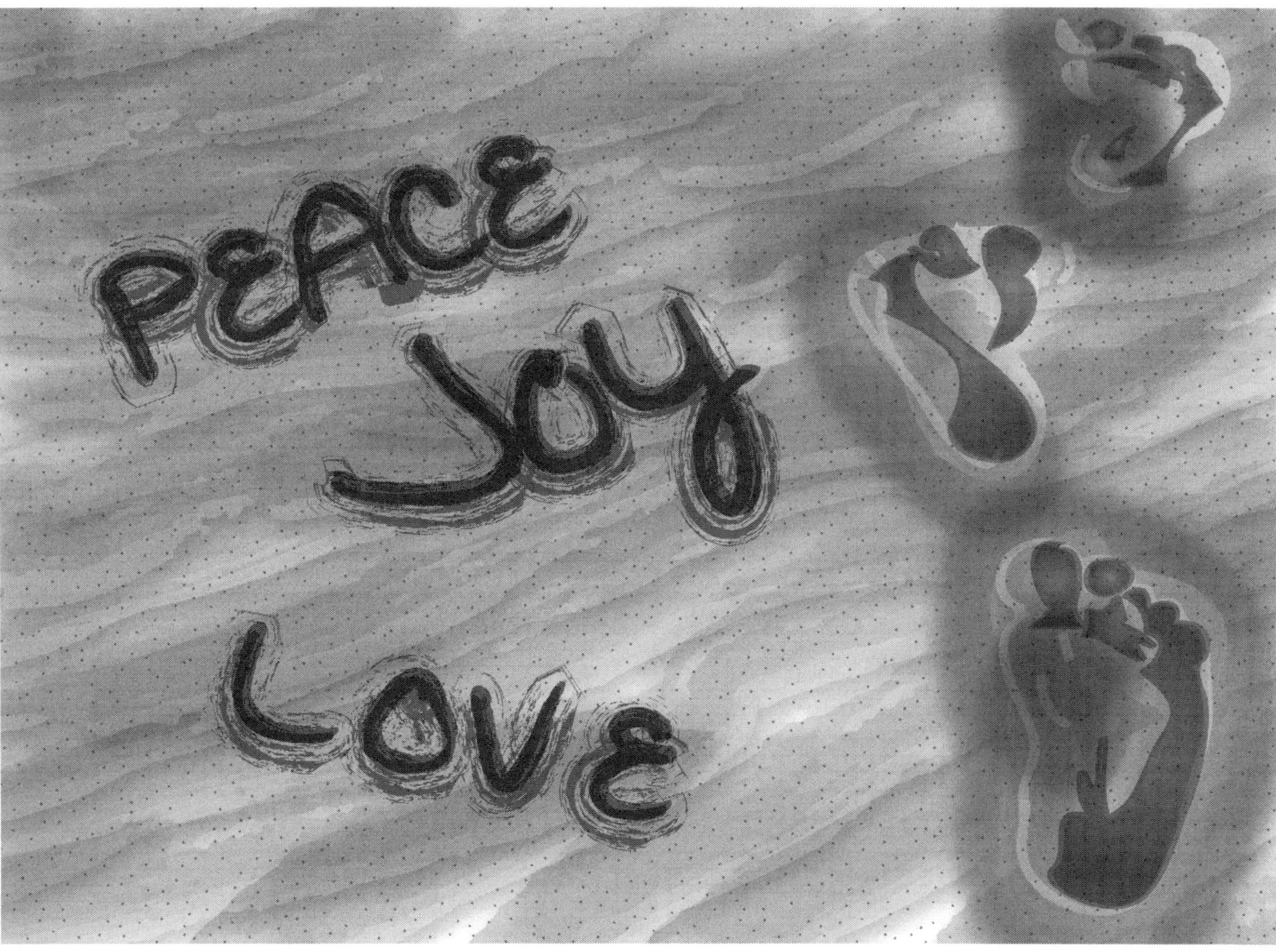
PEACE
JOY
LOVE

The Journey of Another Is None of My Business

I used to wonder why people have to suffer. Even though I had already learned that much of my emotional turmoil was of my own making, this knowledge did not necessarily take away all pain.

Sometimes, just watching others in pain causes emotional distress for me. I want to "fix" them; I want to take away their pain. But now I know if I had the power to take away someone else's pain I would rob them of the dignity of their own journey and, in fact, might cause more pain.

Besides, it is enough work just trying to keep myself fit! I cannot know what is good for anyone else. I can only share how I found out about me and I trust that you have found you somewhere in these pages.

I wish you Peace, Love and Joy on your journey back to you. Namaste.

Acknowledgments

I could have not completed this book without an incredible, amazing group of friends, teachers, mentors, and spiritual guides who have supported me spiritually, emotionally, and in any way they can to keep me on task. I only wish I could name them all. I am profoundly grateful and blessed to have the support from friends Rev. Laura Shackelford, Katrina Bullard, Rev. Mark Accomando, Rev. Dr. Michael J. Kearney, and Dale Olansky, who each in his or her own way inspires me, motivates me, touches my heart, and helps me stay spiritually fit.

Although I dreamed of this writing for many years, Dale was actually the catalyst for the book becoming a reality. Several years ago, Dale heard me share something and insisted I write an article about it and submit it to the daily devotional magazine, Creative Thought. For reasons still unknown to me, I followed her direction, and the article was published.

About a year after the publication of that article, the editor of the magazine contacted me and invited me to write a book. You are holding the results of that connection. Dr. Cynthia Cavalcanti has guided me, counseled me, and mentored me every step of the way from the day of her invitation to this final product. This book would not have happened without the expertise and friendship of Cynthia, whom I cannot thank enough.

I would also like to thank Denise O'Connor, my expert editor, for her awesome work, and Jennifer Forrest, an amazing, insightful, and brilliant artist for the illustrations and cover. Thank you to my friend, Pamela Hower, for sharing with me about how to "shrink it."

A very special acknowledgement and thank you to Rev. Jane Beach for writing the foreword, and to Rev. Dr. Jim Lockhard,Rev. Christian Sorensen D.D., and Dr. Gary Lange for reading the book and writing such beautiful and profound jacket quotes.

Thank you also to Rev. Joe Hooper for always encouraging and supporting me to move forward on my spiritual path, and to Rev. Cynthia James for inspiring me to move beyond my old idea of playing small; your wisdom and passion for truth have changed my life forever.

Made in the USA
San Bernardino, CA
08 June 2014